HERNIA

MESH, MISDIAGNOSIS AND LIFE

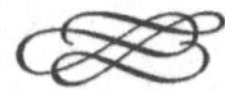

MICHAEL BROOKS

COPYRIGHT AND DISCLAIMER

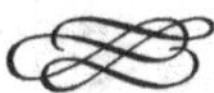

Copyright © Scott M e-commerce All rights reserved.

Disclaimer

All research and clinical material published by Scott M e-commerce is for informational purposes only. Readers are encouraged to confirm the information herein with other sources.The information is not intended to replace medical advice offered by physicians. Scott M e-commerce will not be liable for any direct, indirect, consequential, special, exemplary, or other damages arising therefrom.

DEDICATION

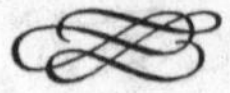

Dedicated to all the people advancing hernia repair surgery and helping people suffer less and live more.

Thank You.

WHAT THIS BOOK CAN DO FOR YOU!

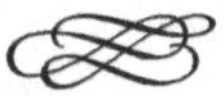

If you have a hernia and you repeatedly do things that hurt you, leave you in discomfort and stop you being able to do the things you want, please read this book from front to back, this is the book I needed when I had my first hernias.

You're not going to be given a way to make all your problems disappear, or do some special technique and see all your pain and injuries go away, its not that type of book.

I'm just going to show you some simple day to day things that can help make life closer to normal again.

. . .

Small changes can make a big difference in your daily life and knowing what not to do is often as important as what to do, so we will cover some of these things.

We are also going to discuss and show examples of some of the options available to people in need of more surgery. Maybe you have been misdiagnosed.

I will try my best to avoid any biases towards any type of repair or idea being pushed currently.

As I am not part of any organisation or industry with emotional or financial gain attached. I hope to show you a detached viewpoint that helps you make rational decisions towards better health.

I am also not against any group or individuals with their own ideas and position within the world of hernias.

At this point there are no perfect fixes to living with and having hernia surgery, you will have to pay a price you don't deserve unfortunately.

. . .

Its, not the Doctors fault, the manufacturers fault, lawyers, journalists or your own, some things have negative consequences no matter how good the intentions of all the people involved.

Please don't despair though, new technologies are being used, recurrence rates are dropping and the future does look better than the past and long may it continue.

No matter what happens in your life, make the best of it. You don't get to decide the hand you're dealt in life but you do get to decide the way you play it.

Take action and use the simple ideas in this book, and try to win back the your joy in life.

MY STORY

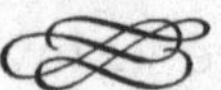

Hi my name is Michael I have been living with hernia's for over 25 years now, I have had 6 hernia's that I know about and 2 operation's both with different technologies. I'm sure I have made every mistake you can make while having hernia's being someone who played sport from childhood and carried on until my mid-twenties.

My life style was the complete opposite of what was needed for long term recovery and avoiding a recurrence. Hopefully you can avoid all the pain, suffering and operations by learning from my experiences.

I had pain in my right groin all the way up to my hip from around 10 years old I never told anyone about this, once I tried but I was not assertive enough about my problem when telling my parents, which was a mistake. You should get checked out as soon as you know something is wrong.

Well as the years went by my pain increased and then one day, I over stretched playing football and it felt like my side had split open, I couldn't ignore the problem anymore.

I ended up having my first hernia operation at 16, at this time the method for fixing hernias was simply to pull the muscle back together and stitch them just like an external wound the problem with this technique is you have a higher chance of a recurrence than today's and previous year's methods.

Also, if it is your first operation do not try to walk too far the day after your op, I tried that and nearly passed out in the toilet it was only 40 feet away, hospital drugs and youthful ignorance, I had them both.

After the operation the Doctor told me it was a double hernia operation and that he had replaced one of my testicles with a prosthesis (false testicle) and that everything had gone well. The reason for taking the testicle was that it didn't always descend totally and was a risk for cancer in my future, if I had the chance to make that decision again I would have risked the cancer later in life rather than listening to the doctor, but that's just me I am not giving anyone advice on that.

Recovering was a slow process for me with my first hernia, I got back to a half decent life one where I was only in pain after exercise but I couldn't push myself as hard without being in agony.

After about a year I decided to go back to see why I was still having trouble, they did another ultra sound scan and couldn't find anything and in the end, I had a CT scan which shows deeper into the body. What they found was that I had 2 more hernias behind the first layer of stomach wall where I had my original operation.

I knew I had to go back for another operation but now I understood why I was in so much pain. If I would have had the CT scan before the first operation, I could have saved myself another operation and whole lot of worrying and pain.

For the second operation they used a new technology a type of hard rigid mesh is placed over the position of the Hernia to hold it in place, apparently it had lowered the recurrence rate to some degree, and after this operation I started to recover fully I could play sports again and lift weights and do all the things I wanted to.

Unfortunately, the story doesn't end there after many years of no virtually no pain I have started to experience pain when I do any sporting activity or heavy lifting. Eventually, I will have to go back for another operation and keep experiencing this, what feels like a never ending story.

In the years that have passed I have learnt many ways to live better with hernias and am hopeful that the new mesh and operating techniques that have become the standard for hernia operations will be a long-term fix to this problem, for me and everyone else experiencing this.

.   .   .

My life dealing with this inconvenience is an inside look for everyone and will hopefully help you avoid a lot of suffering and live a better life.

TYPES OF HERNIAS

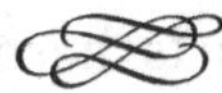

Try making your way through this list and see if there is something that sounds like your hernia or just to find which hernias you don't have.

Just reading through this list will help you get an idea of the vast majority of hernia cases that occur, and this might help you communicate with your doctor or specialist in a way that helps both of you make better decisions.

Inguinal: The most common type of hernia a groin hernia often called Inguinal, this accounts for 70% of all hernias. Intestines push through the inguinal canal, and you get the bump we have all seen with hernias.

Sports:This will be worth the price of the book for some of you, the Sports hernia, its actually not a hernia its an abdominal wall injury. This injury is flat and often unseen. Sports hernia can be mistaken for an inguinal hernia.

Femoral: The Femoral hernia is another groin hernia much like the inguinal, creating a lump in the lower leg or groin. The inguinal canal and femoral canal are where the intestines push through, the femoral type is less common.

Hiatus: These hernias happen when parts of the stomach push up into the chest through the diaphragm. This commonly happens to the over 50's and usually doesn't need to be treated, but always consult your doctor.

Umbilical: A hernia that pushes through the abdominal wall near the belly button. This hernia is usually pain free and can even fix itself over time.

. . .

Epigastric: This hernia occurs between your belly button and your chest bone. These are usually very small hernias but need to be attended to just the same.

Ventral(Incisional): This type of hernia appears if you have an incompletely healed surgical wound.

Spigellian: A hernia through the spigelian fascia a thin membrane similar to a tendon but much thinner. Usually small hernias located on the right side of the groin.

Obturator: This type of hernia occurs more often for women, especially women who have multiple children or older women who have lost a lot of weight. It is a hernia through the pelvic floor, the Obturator opening.

Littres: A littres hernia is the most common congenital groin defect, it is a hernia that occurs between the lower abdomen and the rectum. It happens during congenital pouch formation on the small intestine, that contains tissue left over during the formation of the digestive tract and its organs.

Aymand: The Aymand hernia is a rare hernia where the appendix accompanies the intestines through the opening. A type of hernia which includes the protrusion of the appendix through the inguinal canal is called an Aymand hernia.

DeGarengeots: Much like the Aymand hernia this is when an appendix is part of the hernia. This type would be through the femoral canal.

Richters: The Richter hernia is a hernia of the membrane that attaches the intestine to the abdominal wall of the bowel and protrudes through a fascial (sheet of connective tissue) defect. These are rare but dangerous.

Maydl's: Maydl's hernia is a type of incarcerated hernia popularly known as a hernia in "W" which describes the orientation of the bowel in the hernia sac. Maydl's hernia refers to how the intestines get stuck inside the hernia rather than the position on the body.

Sciatic: A sciatic hernia is a hernia that develops in the pelvic area through the sciatic foramen. It gets its name by being located near the sciatic nerve that runs down from your lower back to the back of your legs. You will probably think of sciatica when you hear this, and this can be one of the symptoms that occurs when the sciatic nerve is pressed on.

Internal: Unlike most hernias, the trapped tissue protrudes inward, rather than outward and as you can imagine is harder to diagnose at first glance. You will not have the expected bulge seen with all external hernias.

These hernias are difficult to identify in women, and being misdiagnosed with endometriosis or idiopathic chronic pelvic pain happens often. One cause of misdiagnosis occurs when the woman lies down flat on an examination table, and the medical signs of the hernia disappear. Knowing this information may help you identify your hernia, by knowing when symptoms disappear.

Perineal: This is a hernia located in your pelvic floor, and usually pushes through on the side of your anus.

In humans this usually occurs after ineffective surgery in the perineal region.

Beclard: a hernia through the opening for the saphenous the large vein that runs up the leg to the femoral vein. This is another type of femoral hernia.

Other types of hernia you can look into if you have not found something that sounds similar to your own:

WHY DID I GET A HERNIA

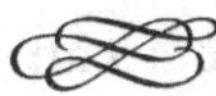

This is a question you have probably asked yourself a bunch of times and heard loads of theories from books, blogs and listening to your friends and families ideas.

The most common theory is usually the genetic flaw you have in your groin, which might be true. This theory has been used because certain families have multiple hernia patients and some have generations of them.

Im not sure if lifestyle is taken into account with the genetic flaw theory, highly sporting families that lift weights and do gardening with a no pain no gain mentality, could make this theory difficult to prove.

On the other hand if families are getting hernias from sneezing and coughing or light exercise the theory would very likely to be true.

Congenital birth defects can cause hernias, this is probably another reason some people think there is a genetic reason for hernias, even though birth defects occur in foetus development and are not hereditary. We know congenital defect do play a part in some hernias particularly the hiatus hernia where the diaphragm connects to the abdomen.

You will likely be told all of the following, you have weak muscles here, tight muscles, loose muscles, you are not stretching enough, your over stretching, you have strength imbalances, you are lifting to much weight, you are lifting asymmetrically, you are twisting to far and so on.

Im sure all of these have some merit in individual cases, with some ideas more or less likely than others.

Weak muscles seems one of the least likely causes when you consider the patient demographics being the highly active athlete. Relatively weak and imbalanced might be a closer diagnosis, even overly tight and strong seems more realistic.

The most common factor across all the ideas is over exercising, this is the worst explanation for all active people that would rather be running around playing sports and spending time in the gym than doing anything else.

It makes me think rest days are probably worth taking more seriously, I would like to see how many hernia patients exercised everyday of the week to see if it is a significant factor.

Hernias seem to occur when explosive movements are needed and turning of the torso is required, add weight lifting or pushing weight into the equation and you have the reason this has happened to a lot of people.

Still it's not a perfect answer, but maybe you have more of an idea what could have happened.

WHAT NOT TO DO WHEN YOU HAVE
A HERNIA

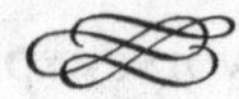

First things first, don't make the obvious mistake of acting like you don't have a gaping hole inside, this can and probably will tear apart even further if not seen t0o.

Don't Lift anything weighing more than you need to, if possible don't lift anything at all. Even if you're extremely strong carrying something relatively light to what you would normally pick up will hurt you, either that day or the next.

If your Hernias are really bad or you're recently back from an operation it's time to not be a gentleman and pick up everyone else's bags. For once in your life you have a real excuse to be the helped not the helper. There is no shame in not helping someone while are terribly injured.

This advice might seem to be obvious but wait a while this is a mistake you're going to make again and again and again; you just forget or you're too polite to not help someone and the next day you pay the price. When moving heavy things use a suit case with wheels if you have to deliver something or take more trips with less in each bag and always get a shopping trolley instead of a basket. <u>Don't worry about what other people think</u>, everyone is too concerned with their own lives to worry about what you're doing.

Cut down on sex if your partner has a high sex drive, I would have a chat with her about lowering the frequency of sex you have every week and try to spread it out, no weekend marathon's if you can help it. If you have sex for hours on end then maybe the duration will have to be sacrificed. In the end it's up to you but you will experience some consequences of pain after. Of course, this advice is for when your hernias are bad or after your operation and during recovery. It would be best not to have sex at all for the first weeks after an operation, if you can help it.

. . .

If you need to use the restroom go right away rather than holding it for an extended time period, this mistake consistently leads to pain.

Don't strain yourself on the toilet just wait as long as you can it will save you a lot of pain if you don't try to strain. Buy a book if you have to and get a high fibre diet, you don't want to be constipated as well. And try not to wipe yourself too hard if your hernias are in your groin it does not help.

You will not hear this embarrassing advice in a pamphlet.

STRANGULATED HERNIA

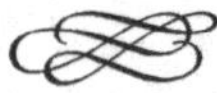

The strangulated hernia, the number one thing you need to think about avoiding when you have a hernia.

A strangulated hernia is when your intestines get clamped down between your abdominal muscles cutting of your blood supply.

Other hernia related occurrences can leave you with all types of problems, but the strangulated hernia can kill you.

The number one thing you can do to avoid getting a strangulated hernia is consult your doctor, and arrange a surgery to fix your hernia as soon as possible. The longer you have your hernia unfixed, the longer you have to be unlucky and have a strangulation.

Strangulation of the hernia is rare, but it happens and sometimes people die from this.

Some of the symptoms include, fever, vomiting, nausea, high levels of pain, the bulge becoming a dark, red or purple colour and not being able to pass wind or make a bowel movement.

This is unlikely to happen to you, but it's better to be aware of this rather than being unaware and too slow to take action.

SPORTS HERNIA

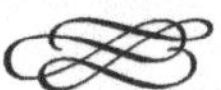

What is a Sports Hernia? And why you have to know.

The hernia that is not visible and does not present with the bump so common with most hernias.

It is actually not considered to be a hernia, the real name for it is athletic pubalgia, a tear in the muscle or tendon of the groin.

This type of hernia is difficult to detect and often misdiagnosed as an inguinal hernia which can lead to unnecessary suffering if the incorrect surgery is performed.

The sports hernia is most common amongst soccer players and other sports with twisting and turning at high speed, kicking and other explosive movements.

Some tears can heal themselves or be managed with anti inflammatories and physio therapy with differing levels of success.

The strange nature of this type of hernia is that it can go away, then reoccur when doing any physical activity. Pain, discomfort and an injury type response to sports and lifting can happen in a very predictable sequence, work out, pain, recover from injury, repeat.

If you're in a situation where the tear is so bad it effects your life on a daily basis and stops you doing all the things you want to do, you will have to try surgery to fix the tear.

If pain continues after the healing process should have resolved everything, go back to your doctor and discuss it. They might suggest a second surgery called an adductor tenotomy, this procedure helps give your tendon some more slack by lengthening the tendon by making an incision.

I hope you can tell which type of hernia you have after reading this, as it might save you a lot of trouble in the future.

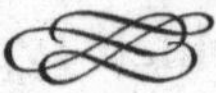

Wether you have temporary or long term pain you will have to deal with it in some way.

You might be lucky enough to be able to bear your pain or even just take the occasional paracetamol to help numb the pain. Unfortunately for a lot of hernia patients the pain does persist and is painful enough to get in the way of work and all other activities you need to perform.

How you deal with your pain is an important thing to contemplate, the way pain management is handled by some can be even more damaging than the pain.

Most pain relieving drugs are part of the opioid family, these drugs can become highly addictive and if you have to pay for them yourself they can be expensive.

Opioids are the first thing that will be given to you because they work, they are not perfect solutions but they do work. They work temporarily and in countries where the strongest opioids can be administered to patients this can cause all sorts of problems.

The opioids are getting people addicted to all types of pain killers at a price the patient cannot afford, the patient then looks into finding alternatives with many turning to the black market for their opium fix, which is usually heroin.

Im not suggesting that you don't use opioids for pain, but I am suggesting you at least try other methods that might help you in the long term without the need for ever stronger pills.

. . .

Just being aware that addictions to seemingly harmless substances can lead you down a bad road, could save you from a world of pain.

Lets talk about some of the other ways of relieving pain, I can't list all of them now but here are some of the most commonly used methods and some that have good results.

Light exercise that doesn't hurt your hernia. It does seem counter intuitive to do more of the activity that may have helped put you in this position but exercise creates the release of endorphins which helps improve mood and blocks pain signals. You will have to find an exercise that does not effect your hernia, something like swimming or cycling once you are able, could be an option.

Tens units are becoming a popular solution for pain, tens stand for transcutaneous electrical nerve stimulation, these devices send electrical pulses through the skin to help subdue the pain. I have not tried this but have heard good things, it's worth a try.

.   .   .

Physiotherapy kind of ties into the light exercise method, but your guided by a professional that will help you find the right exercises and routines so you do not over or under exercise your muscles. If you have access to this option and you are willing to maintain the practices it should help to some degree, even if the pain doesn't dissipate it might help you find your physical boundaries sooner and strengthen your weaknesses.

If you have tried everything and you really need to do something immediately you could try talking to your doctor about nerve injections or even having a neurectomy to severe or remove the nerves in a surgery. The neurectomy is a last resort type of treatment, I would never recommend unnecessary surgery, not even for vanities sake.

Whatever you choose to do, make sure you seek medical advice and make sure to do something rather than nothing.

BATHING AND CLEANING

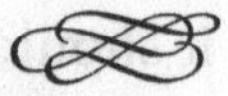

*I*f you're a bath person who loves to just lay there for hours and relax and just let all the tension and stress of the day fade away falling half asleep in a haze of steam, and the smell of oils and aromatic candles. Sorry my friend you're going to have to change to showers or at least just have warm baths and not stay in it long at all as it makes your hernia feel weak, it's a horrible feeling. Try doing your usual thing but to a lesser extent and see how it feels to you, everyone is different so literally test the waters.

I prefer to have some tension in the muscles around the hernia but that might be a personal preference rather than something that works in general.

· · ·

You should have paperwork telling you the best way to take care of and clean your wounds after the operation.

For all people who have just had operations the shower is a lot easier as you don't have lie down in it. Don't stand in the shower too long if your only a few of days out, you will still be weak from your operation your probably better off to just wash with a cloth sitting down.

Remember to make sure you have clean hand's any time you touch near your wound after an operation, infection can lead to even more problem's.

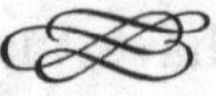

nother task made difficult and painful, especially right after you have had your operation.

You should have some advice from your hospital about how long it will be until you can start driving again. Some will tell you to start driving again after a week and some will tell you to take a month or more.

You can't really change the advice you get concerning when to start driving, but you can change some of the little things you will do when you get back to driving.

· · ·

Hopefully your pain should be light enough for you to move without restriction and your medication should not be effecting you're ruction time and consciousness. That should be obvious but someone is going to drive before they are ready and drive around full of strong pain killers, its not worth the risk.

If you do get into an accident straight after an operation your insurance might be invalidated. Some insurance companies do not insure people for weeks after an operation, so look into your insurer to see if you're covered.

Not only that you are asking for all sorts of legal problems if you hurt someone while driving medicated, and being asked by medical professionals not to drive for a specific time period. Your sentencing may be increased if you are shown to be negligent.

Your licensing agency might need notifying depending on the type of license you have. Especially if you are employed in a profession that requires you to drive continuously with multiple passengers or drive large vehicles that require you to have different licenses.

Its worth practising all the possible motions you will have to perform while driving when sitting in a stationary position, rather than finding out how you feel while in motion. Adjust your seat so you don't overstretch and take it slow at first. No cross country road trips is probably a good idea.

Don't take this information lightly, this is probably the most dangerous moment in your whole journey back to recovery.

EXERCISE ADVICE

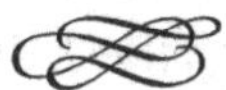

This is a difficult thing to deal with for almost all active hernia sufferers, especially when you consider some type of exercise might have helped lead to the injury in the first place.

It's very hard to exercise without engaging your core, some exercises engage the core more than others and some create unneeded imbalances while being performed.

Anything that encourages twisting, turning and explosive movements has a higher chance of sports type hernias occurring or being effected.

· · ·

In the weight room you will have to take it easy and lift light until you have recovered fully.

Breathing out when lifting and not having the habit of keeping a solid air filled stomach might be the best thing you ever learn to do, when it comes to avoiding more hernias that is.

Sometimes you will need your core to hold or pull you up so breathing out a lot will not be possible. Its good to know if you feel pressure on your stomach when lifting you can just breathe out and reduce some of the pressure.

Some say the worst exercise you can do to create a hernia is the one armed row on a bench. The unnecessary leg position being a factor, with one knee on the bench and one on the floor and stretching out your groin area, also just the fact you're using a one armed row rather than a bar adds extra pressure on your groin.

The asymmetry of certain exercises only adds to the pressure on your abdomen so be careful and consider this when choosing your exercises based on the health of your core.

The sport that creates the most hernias is football (soccer) the worlds most popular sport, the pressure as you hit a solid object while elevating one leg and thrusting your hip to get maximum power, often at a stretch all adds to up to groin troubles.

Sports similar to football will likely give similar results. Just another thing to consider when choosing activities.

Getting advice from a physiotherapist about safer options can help you avoid injury, progressively improve your condition and help you not to cause more damage than necessary. A tailored approach from a good physiotherapist could save you a lot of trouble in the long run.

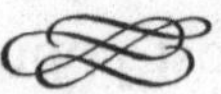

With this section its really up to you to decide what you feel comfortable wearing the most I can tell you is that I like to just wear boxers with an elasticated waist like a Calvin Klein style boxer short so it supports where my hernia is. I absolutely hate jock straps and wouldn't recommend them myself but again this is your choice my only suggestion is that you try all the options for yourself.

The first thing they will give you to wear out of the hospital is the Jock Strap which as a man I can really say I hate the thing, maybe it's perfect for women I can see this should work. But from my perspective it's a male genitalia strangulation device. I don't want to steer anyone wrong so at least try it; I just don't like it.

You can now purchase something called a hernia belt inguinal truss support I have never tried one of these but a lot of people seem to really find this helps. They are supposed to be a good prevention to stop your hernia from popping out as well.

If you have an umbilical hernia which, as you have guessed is where your belly button is you can acquire an umbilical hernia belt it's a kind of strap that holds you in place.

And last but not least the boxer shorts with elasticated waist, also y fronts with the same waist exist if you prefer them.

Always consult a doctor about anything of this nature. The type of Hernia, position and possibility of a strangulated/incarcerated Hernia is something to take into consideration.

. . .

A strangulated Hernia is when a Hernia gets trapped on the outside of the stomach wall, this is very dangerous and requires immediate medical attention.

LOSING A TESTICLE

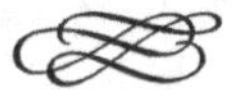

*L*osing a testicle doesn't happen to every Hernia sufferer, but it happens to a lot of people who have Hernias in their groin region.

Most people wonder if you are still fertile if you lose a testicle, the answer is yes! Also most people don't know that people with 2 testicles can only orgasm from one testicle at a time, so it really doesn't change much fertility wise.

You will be asked if you would like a false testicle to replace the original, that is what I did and I think it was the right decision 15 years later. The false testicle doesn't hang low like the other testicle when you're not aroused so it can look a little weird to you at times, but when you are aroused it should line up and look almost as it would if you had your original testicle, and really that's the only time anyone should be looking at your testicles anyway.

Losing one testicle does not affect your testosterone level much although it does vary from person to person, if you lose both testicles you may have to have testosterone replacement of some kind, you should seek medical advice for this as it is different for each person, as you can imagine with dosage and age factor's varying.

Low testosterone in males can lead to side effects such as low muscle development and the growth of breast tissue on top of the male's chest, I tell you these thing's so that you make sure you deal with it and make sure to get the proper advice and medicate if need be.

I have had one side effect of losing a testicle and not a very nice one, they call it an oscillating testicle it only happens to me about once a year but it is horrible, the testicle changes angle in the scrotum and can be totally vertical, if this happens to you try not to

panic go to the toilet if you can, and don't manipu-
late your testicle in any way, make yourself relax and
stay in a seated position if you can, with your geni-
tals hanging freely.

This can last for me a couple of hours at a time I
won't go anywhere when this happens. It is not
painful but looking at it can make you feel nauseous
as I cannot tell which way my testicle has moved to
get into that position. Do not mistake this for a
testicular torsion where you will be in pain and need
to most likely have surgery and have the testicle
removed, a doctor might jump to this conclusion if
they are not informed. An oscillating testicle occurs
because of scar tissue in the scrotum and can happen
at any time so be careful if it happens to you.

PARTIALLY ABLED

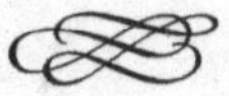

You're not disabled and you don't have the look of a man/woman that is injured.

Some hernias don't even come with a bump, they are almost completely flat but the muscle has still torn inside.

Guess what everyone thinks about your injuries? Over exaggerated and just the same as a small injury or operation they have. You cannot expect other people to understand, most people will not consider that your body is ripped open from the inside and all your nerves are damaged.

· · ·

Everyone judges a book by its cover whether we like it or not, when you see the beautiful people or wealthy people you don't consider the problem's they have just like you.

It's the same with hernias that are not immediately visible, you're going to be met with a level of scepticism at times even though you're actually only a partially abled person living in pain and discomfort.

Things like helping someone push a car to get it started can be awkward, when you turn down the offer to help it might not be taken well.

Saying you had an operation recently can help you get out of situations that your body might not be able to handle, so keep that in your tool box of canned answers to protect yourself from injury.

CHANGE YOUR LIFE OR BE FRUSTRATED

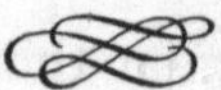

You can fight or accept things in your mind, but the material world doesn't care about your thoughts and feelings. You need to find out what your new boundaries are and reassess them, now and in the future as your injuries change and your options open and close.

Your sports, hobbies, fitness and exercise regimes will have to be reconsidered, especially if they push your body to its limits.

Unfortunately, your goals might have to change and this might be hard for you to accept.

. . .

I completely changed my life from one of endless sports and training in the gym, to reading, learning and trying to make money through investments and business, I didn't see that coming.

At first the changes can be depressing, what you lose from your past life can be massive but you do gain the chance to live a completely different life.

Another life, with new dreams and ambitions to work towards. Whole new worlds can open up to you when looking into things that you had no interest in originally.

Try to do the things you have always loved if you can, but if you can't do those things don't worry it's a big wide world full of interesting experiences and the vacuum left by your past will be filled with new things that will lead to your next big adventure.

MULTIPLE OPERATIONS

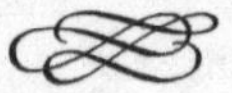

If you are going back for your second or third operation make sure to take your recovery as seriously as you ever have, I would say the more operations you have the more careful you need to be.

Your tissue becomes weaker with each operation that is performed on the same spot as the previous operation was. Your healing capabilities may decrease with age as well.

Speak to your doctor about the likelihood of a successful surgery and make a decision from there.

. . .

My surgeon warned me not to have another surgery as my tissue would be weak from my previous operations despite me only being in my 30's.

It is just another thing to consider unfortunately.

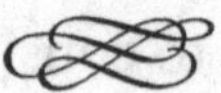

What is a mesh? A mesh is a biological or synthetic patch or plug made to cover the hole in your abdominal wall and add structural strength so recurrence of injury is less likely to occur.

Why do most surgeons prefer to use mesh? Mesh has proven to lower the recurrence rate of having another hernia significantly. That is in the short and long term.

Each type of hernia surgery is slightly different, so statistics vary for each surgery that uses mesh. And meshes have improved over time becoming more flexible, and many other factors of improvement have occurred, even the choice to use different meshes to fit the individual needs of the patient e.g. one patient might need a thicker stronger mesh than another person with a smaller hernia, the person with the smaller hernia can have a thinner lighter mesh which has the advantage of causing less inflammation.

I will not quote the statistics but I promise you, recurrence rates are much lower than non mesh surgeries and are different for each type of operation.

What are the different types of mesh available?

Synthetic : Hernia mesh made of synthetic materials come in woven or non-woven sheets. The synthetic materials can be absorbable, non-absorbable or a combination of both. The most popular types of surgical mesh are made from polypropylene – a synthetic plastic.

Biologics : Biologic mesh (or bio mesh) is a type of surgical mesh made from an organic biomaterial (such as porcine dermis, porcine small intestine submucosa, bovine dermis or pericardium, and the dermis or fascia lata of a cadaveric human).

Bio Absorbable Mesh : Absorbable mesh degrades and loses strength over time. It is not used to provide long-term reinforcement to the repaired hernia.

Patches and plugs : The most popular type of mesh is just a type of patch that is fixed over the wound, there is another type called the plug which is a 2 part mesh including a patch with a circular whole which is made to house the second part of the mesh which fills the hole.

NON MESH REPAIR

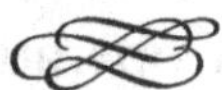

Getting your hernia fixed without the mesh has its pros and cons just like the mesh repair does. The choice of repair should be contemplated as each situation is different, each patient has different needs and the doctor has to consider multiple factors.

Having a mesh repair as a growing child could result in more pain than is necessary therefore the repair without mesh should be considered.

The likelihood of having another hernia is increased by not using the mesh technique but non mesh surgeries have less chance of complications as there is no foreign body left inside the patient.

You have to weigh up your options, the chances of having complications from your mesh operation are low but a complication can be more serious than having another hernia operation some time in the future.

I would hope you look up the statistics for your particular type of operation and the chances of complication then see if you want to add extra risk of complications rather than only worry about decreasing the chances of having another hernia operation.

There are multiple ways to perform a non mesh repair, the most popular types of surgeries are called the Bassini, the McVay, Desarda, Lichtenstein and the Shouldice. You can look into each type but the consensus seems to be that the shouldice technique has the best results without using mesh.

The only problem with the Shouldice style of repair is that not every surgeon can do this, and if you don't ask your consultant what type of surgery they do, you might end up with some other technique and more than likely a simple mesh fix will be offered first.

The other non mesh repairs are still very good and should not just be dismissed. Some surgeons have high success rates with the surgery they are most comfortable with and have performed repeatedly.

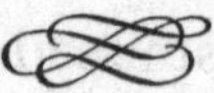

Removing mesh can help many people suffering from the complications that can an occur from using mesh in a small percentage of people.

This is not recommended for everyone with a little bit of pain and discomfort from their hernia operation, that is to be expected unfortunately.

Removing mesh is not the easiest thing a surgeon can do, and will not be the correct course of action for every patient.

. . .

The reason there is difficulty removing the mesh is because the mesh becomes embedded within the tissue and is completely submerged. Removal means the surgeon has to cut away the mesh while trying to leave you as much tissue remaining as possible.

Some mesh may have to be left inside due to becoming attached where it's difficult for the surgeon to remove or another consideration such as a piece of mesh not causing any harm.

Even with the difficult task of getting every bit of your mesh out, surgeons do have success with this procedure and lots of patients turn their life around.

RECURRENCE VERSUS COMPLICATIONS

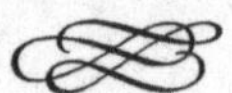

Your choice of operations is limited and really comes down to 2 choices, use a mesh repair and have a small chance of complications or have a non mesh repair which gives you a higher chance of coming back for a hernia operation.

I hope the information that you obtain from this book helps you speak to consultants and surgeons in a rational manner so you can find the right option for your unique situation.

Your work, lifestyle, age and health may be factors that influence your decisions and the guidance you are given by health practitioners. The actual hernia will be a determining factor, the size being the most obvious differential.

THE POSSIBLE COMPLICATIONS

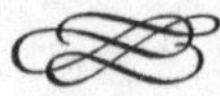

I'm not looking to scare you or give you a false perspective about the success and failure of hernia operations but I'm also not going to hold back and leave you in the dark about some of the horrible thing that have happened to people.

Most hernia operations have great outcomes and the complications that can occur only effect a small minority of the millions of patients around the world.

The majority of mesh patches resemble a rectangular or oval shape and the structure closely resembles a fishing net with very tiny holes where water would pour through. As brilliant as. some of the designs are they almost all have faults, some much worse than others and the previous generations meshes that have been banned are hardly worth mentioning.

The worst of the worst have stopped being produced, they had metal in the centre of the mesh leading to terrible infections and all the terrible consequences you can imagine, including death.

Well that's made you feel better hasn't it.

The most common complaint with hernias is pain and chronic pain, here are some of the horrible reasons why this occurs more often when using a mesh.

We just talked about how the mesh resembles a fishing net, well one of the downsides to this is, as your mesh starts to merge with your tissue your nerve endings end up intertwined with the mesh, they can get entangled, stretched and over time the mesh can shrink to almost 50% of its original size and even break inside you as it becomes hard and brittle. Some kind of ball up, like its being crumpled up. Not only this but the edges can become very sharp, sharp enough to cut your surgeons fingers when being removed.

With the nerves being entrapped and the mesh folding back in on it self while attached to your tissues its no wonder why so many people have some type of long term pain, wether it's chronic or not.

Adhesions can be a problem, the mesh becoming attached to the bowel which can lead to all sorts of problems and just as bad if not worse some have had the mesh attach to the spermatic cord and damage it to the point of sexual disfunction and the loss of a testicle.

Other mesh complications include, severe inflammation, fistulas, abscesses and infections.

THE FUTURE

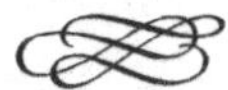

The future of medicine looks like a future of miracles with stem cell bringing new healing abilities to humanity which were the stuff of science fiction not so long age.

Gene editing as a prevention to many if not all hereditary flaws in our genome allowing hernia sufferers with a genetic predisposition for hernias to help their children stop the cycle of suffering.

For people with chronic pain there might be some hope now scientists are studying what makes people born feeling no pain at all the way they are. With the help of gene manipulation this could be a great advance for all the people suffering in this way.

. . .

The future does look bright so no matter what you do never give up and never give up on hope for your future and the future of you progeny.

FINALLY

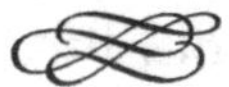

*P*lease consult your doctor and give them all the information you have concerning your problems. Never hold back information about yourself that you think might be relevant, so your doctor can make the most informed decision for solving your issues.

Time's change and so with technological advancement we can see a future where hernias will be seen as a problem of the past.

Make sure to live your life to the fullest you can, we are all given a different set of cards to play throughout our lives, so enjoy them and play them well.

You may have to adapt to your bodies weaknesses unexpectedly, this can be frustrating, but you will strengthen in other way's and find new strengths and interests to fulfil your life.

No great story was told without a struggle against adversity.

Always consult a doctor with your medical problem's, a specialist if possible.

Thanks for your time I wish you the greatest luck in the adventure which is your life.

Michael Brooks

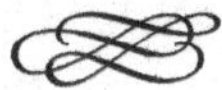

*T*hank you for reading this far.

Please leave an honest review if you have the time.

Hopefully this helps you navigate your hernia journey with a little less suffering and gives you some hope for your future.

Good luck and good health to you.

Thanks again

. . .